A DERMATOLOGIST'S LITTLE INSTRUCTION BOOK

Dr. Robert A. Norman

QMP

Quality Medical Publishing, Inc.

ST. LOUIS, MISSOURI

1999

It is the responsibility of the individual practitioner to evaluate the applicability or appropriateness of any particular opinion or advice in the context of the actual clinical or personal situation and with all due consideration given to new information, research, or developments. The authors, contributors, and publisher assume no liability for any real or potential damages resulting from the use of the information and opinions contained herein.

Printed in the United States of America

Quality Medical Publishing, Inc.
11970 Borman Drive, Suite 222
St. Louis, Missouri 63146
Telephone: 1-800-423-6865
Web site: http://www.qmp.com

ISBN 1-57626-126-3

For all those
who have been my teachers—
physicians, patients, friends,
and family

ACKNOWLEDGMENTS

The concept and source of inspiration for this book came from Dr. Daniel J. Waters, the author of *A Heart Surgeon's Little Instruction Book,* and *A Surgeon's Little Instruction Book*. I am grateful to Dr. Waters for allowing me to include in this volume some of my favorite quotes and pearls previously published in these *Little Instruction* books.

Many thanks to James Fitzpatrick, M.D., John Aeling, M.D., Rob Albergo, M.D., Charles Perakis, D.O., and Dennis Miller.

If you have clinical pearls that you would like to include for the next edition of this book, please send them to me in care of Quality Medical Publishing, Inc.

Dr. Robert A. Norman

March 1999

CONTENTS

Diagnosis 1-78

Treatment and Results 79-155

Patients and Their Families 156-205

Staff and Colleagues. 206-240

Professional Development 241-317

Personal Development 318-343

Diagnosis

It should be the function of medicine to have people die young as late as possible.

Ernst L. Wynder, M.D.

1. Always conduct a complete examination; avoid moving directly to the easy and obvious conclusion.

2. Order all reasonable tests to confirm the final diagnosis and rule out the differential diagnoses.

3. Seek a consulting opinion when involved in an area outside of your knowledge, skill, or experience.

4. If you are unhappy with the quality of a diagnostic study, your patient deserves to have the study repeated.

5. Never guess when you can know.

6. Never discourage a patient who wants a second opinion.

Doctors are busy playing God when so few of us have the qualifications. And besides, the job is taken.

Bernie S. Siegel, M.D.

7. If you read your own slides, keep your glasses and microscope clean.

8. Use a magnifying glass or loops to examine the skin. Patients are more impressed than when you use only the naked eye.

9. Obtain a second opinion on all dark and irregularly pigmented lesions.

10. When your patient with a rash complains of a recent sore throat, look for guttate psoriasis; it often looks like a scattering of off-white, small, drop-like papules and plaques.

11. *Question:* What's the difference between a rash and an eruption?

Answer: The cost of a consultation fee.

12. In any patient with a generalized rash and lymphadenopathy, check the soles and test for syphilis.

13. Beware of trichorrhexis nodosa in African-American women if they are using chemical hair relaxers and complain that their hair falls out or won't grow.

14. If you suspect malignancy, make certain you get a biopsy before performing electrodessication.

15. "When in doubt, cut it out." Perform a biopsy when you're not sure what something is.

16. You can learn more from one mistake than from a dozen triumphs.

17. Work-related skin disease represents one of the largest percentages of occupational illnesses, the most commonly occurring being irritant contact dermatitis.

18. A history of childhood eczema is the most important predictive factor for the development of adult hand dermatitis; a history of atopic dermatitis is a significant risk factor for occupational skin disease.

19. Any chronic eczematous lesion on the areola or nipple that is unresponsive to treatment with topical corticosteroids should be evaluated by excisional biopsy.

20. Look for signs of insulin resistance in a patient with acanthosis nigricans.

21. Diabetic patients are susceptible to severe and frequent bacterial infections.

22. Check the feet of all patients with diabetes—diabetic ulcers and other diabetes-related disorders are enormous health problems.

23. Screen all patients with recurrent cutaneous candidiasis for diabetes.

24. Vitiligo can occur in patients with insulin-dependent diabetes, hypothyroidism, and Addison's disease.

25. Acanthosis nigricans is associated with obesity, diabetes, and use of systemic steroids, niacin, estrogen, pituitary extract, and testosterone.

26. Erythema nodosum (a form of panniculitis) is most commonly associated with the use of oral contraceptives and with streptococcal infections.

27. Always remember *CSD*—*c*olor, *s*hape, and *d*istribution—when evaluating any skin disorder.

28. When you find an anesthetic area of leukoderma, always think of Hansen's disease.

29. If dark pigment develops in a single nail of a person aged 50 to 80 years of age, rule out melanoma.

30. Always look at a patient's eyes. If the patient has blue eyes, think melanoma—not pigmented basal cell carcinoma.

31. Rule out melanoma if any band in the nail is wider at the base or darkening.

32. Acral lentiginous melanoma is the most common melanoma type among Japanese, African-Americans, Hispanics, and Native Americans.

33. The leaching of pigment into the surrounding nail-fold—Hutchinson's sign—is pathognomonic for melanoma.

34. Melanomas can appear on any body part, but the primary tumors most commonly occur on the lower extremity in women and the trunk in men.

35. Make certain that as many of your patients as possible know the four basic warning signs of melanoma: *ABCD*—*a*symmetry (the two sides don't match), *b*order (irregular), *c*olor (variety of shades), and *d*iameter (larger than ¼ inch).

36. Promote the concept of self-examination. Remember the Skin Cancer Foundation's slogan—"Skin cancer: If you can spot it, you can stop it."

37. Telogen effluvium can be found in a patient with severe illness, such as metastatic cancer, or after the patient has undergone a major surgical procedure.

38. Telogen effluvium most commonly occurs in women 3 months after giving birth.

39. All patients for whom oral retinoid therapy is prescribed should receive pretreatment counseling about potential side effects. They should also undergo pretreatment blood lipid and liver function studies, and a complete blood cell count should be performed.

40. In all patients with persistent scaly patches that respond poorly to topical therapy, consider mycosis fungoides.

41. All female patients of child-bearing age for whom oral isotretinoin therapy is prescribed should first undergo a serum pregnancy test within 2 weeks before starting treatment. If the results of the pregnancy test are negative, they should be given the consent forms to sign and be instructed that they should begin taking isotretinoin on the second or third day of their next normal menstrual period.

42. Herpes gestationis is an autoimmune disorder that usually begins in the late second trimester, is *not* related to herpes virus infection, and commonly recurs in subsequent pregnancy.

43. Pruritic urticarial papules and plaques of pregnancy (PUPPP) usually begin in the third trimester, are much more common than herpes gestationis, and usually do not recur in subsequent pregnancy.

44. Note the pigmentary changes that occur in a normal pregnancy—melasma, linea nigra, hyperpigmentation of the axillae, inner thighs, nipples, areolae, and anogenital area, and darkening of nevi and ephelides.

45. Nearly 85% of persons 12 to 25 years of age will have some acne lesions.

46. The most prevalent skin disease in pediatric patients is acne vulgaris. The neonatal and adolescent periods are the two peaks of onset.

47. A "rash" on the face, chest, and back (with no prior history of the same) on a 32-year-old patient can still be acne.

48. About 10% of scalp hairs are in the telogen (preshedding) phase at any given time.

49. When hair loss and alopecia are present, don't forget to ask about nervous habits and pulling the hair out.

50. Twenty-five percent of patients with scabies may be affected with *Staphylococcus aureus*.

51. In any patient with a skin eruption of increased severity, atypical appearance, or resistance to treatment, think of AIDS.

52. *Staphylococcus aureus* is the most common cutaneous bacterial pathogen in HIV disease, most commonly presenting as superficial folliculitis.

53. Although decreasing in incidence, Kaposi's sarcoma is the most common cutaneous malignancy in HIV disease.

54. In HIV-positive patients, look for bacterial infections *(S. aureus),* fungal infections (mucocutaneous candidiasis and dermatophytosis), and viral infections (condyloma, common and plantar warts, herpes, varicella zoster, molluscum contagiosum, and Epstein-Barr virus).

55. Several studies have shown a prevalence of skin disease in more than 90% of HIV-infected patients.

56. The most common cutaneous manifestations of HIV infection are papulosquamous dermatoses, including seborrheic dermatitis and xerosis.

57. Remember the four *D*'s of pellagra—diarrhea, dermatitis, dementia, and death—and that niacin deficiency is most common in alcoholics.

58. When diagnosing insect bites, look for three lesions clustered together, known as "breakfast, lunch, and dinner"—the insect's meals, that is.

59. A *scar* represents excess collagen deposition at the site of a healing wound, which does not extend beyond the limits of the original trauma.

60. A *keloid* represents excessive collagen deposition at the site of a healing wound, which generally grows beyond the bounds of the original trauma.

61. Xanthelasma is usually not associated with elevated serum triglyceride levels.

62. Urticaria, hand dermatitis, and erythema nodosum can be types of dermatophytid reactions from tinea pedis.

63. When your patient is a child, get down to his or her level and talk.

64. With all pediatric patients exhibiting unusual bruising, abrasions, burns, dermatitis, traumatic alopecia, or any irregular cutaneous patterns, consider the possibility of child abuse.

65. Any prepubertal child with scaly scalp dermatitis or seborrheic dermatitis should be considered to have a dermatophyte infection until proven otherwise.

66. The most common cause of endemic tinea capitis is *Trichophyton tonsurans.*

67. Any child who presents with a scalp abscess should be considered to have a kerion.

68. A circular scaly or crusted bald spot on the scalp of an African-American child should be considered tinea capitis until proven otherwise.

69. With acquired circumscribed hair loss in children, consider alopecia areata, tinea capitis, and trichotillomania.

70. Almost all infants will develop telogen effluvium during the first 6 months of life; many babies have more hair at birth than at 3 or 4 months of age.

71. Typically, atopic dermatitis initially appears in infants between 1 and 4 months of age.

72. More than 90% of the people who develop atopic dermatitis will have manifested the disease by adolescence, and by that age they will no longer have symptoms of atopic dermatitis.

73. If diaper dermatitis is present for more than 3 days, you can expect it to be superinfected by *Candida albicans.*

74. The most common cutaneous bacterial infection in children is impetigo, caused by streptococci, staphylococci, or a combination of the two organisms.

75. When you observe children with keratotic papules on the face, outer upper arms, and thighs, consider keratosis pilaris and ask whether other family members have had the same disorder.

76. To make the diagnosis of scabies, look for infestation of the areola and nipples in females and the penis in males.

77. Look in the mouth and check the nails of patients you suspect have lichen planus; it helps make the diagnosis.

78. Never let a published scientific article stand in the way of common sense.

Experience is what we call the accumulation of our mistakes.

Yiddish folk saying

TREATMENT AND RESULTS

If you want truly to understand something, try to change it.

Kurt Lewin

Wrinkles should merely indicate where the smiles have been.

Mark Twain

79. The basic principle of dermatology is, "If it's wet, dry it. If it's dry, wet it."

80. All your patients should look younger by their third visit.

81. Base your clinical decisions on science, not advertising.

82. Be circumspect when you dismiss new ideas or new technology.

83. Never forget that even minor procedures can have major complications.

84. Don't panic—even when it is obviously the most rational thing to do.

85. Making a procedure more complex doesn't necessarily make it better.

86. During a long surgical procedure, soothe your nerves with relaxing music.

87. Avoid out-of-body experiences while doing your major cases.

88. Don't worry about being fast—worry about being effective.

89. Never throw instruments.

90. Tell acne patients being treated to expect a possible exacerbation of acne vulgaris, representing an externalization of deep-seated acne lesions.

91. Consider the use of glycolics with all acne patients.

92. Tell all acne patients that they may not see beneficial effects for the first 6 weeks of therapy.

93. Acne treatment failures most commonly result from the physician's not instructing the patient about the proper application of medications or providing information about the length of time for maximum improvement (6 months or more) and a clear picture of expected results.

94. Don't be *afraid* to perform a new procedure, just be *prepared.*

95. There are land mines in even the most routine cases.

96. Technology is sometimes more advanced than our ability to apply it properly.

97. Be suspicious of procedures that are "hyped" to the general public before they have been proved to be advantageous or beneficial.

98. Although tretinoin cream works to decrease wrinkling and irregular pigmentation of photoaged skin, it is not a panacea, and you should emphasize to all patients that they should limit sun exposure and use sunscreens.

99. Tell a patient to always try a new skin care product on his or her inner arm before applying it to the face. This area is the most sensitive. If you can tolerate it on the inner arm without a problem, you are ready to try it on your face.

100. Consider Moh's surgery to treat aggressive facial cancers or recurrent skin cancers in areas in which maximum preservation of normal tissue is crucial.

101. All pigment lasers are expensive, and patients risk hypopigmentation, hyperpigmentation, and scarring.

102. Remember that laser surgery is still surgery.

103. Never use a laser instrument when less expensive techniques are available that work equally well.

104. Laser stands for *l*ight *a*mplification by the *s*timulated *e*mission of *r*adiation—not *l*atest *a*dvanced *s*ource of *e*xtra *r*emuneration.

105. When using a carbon dioxide laser, protect your eyes, use adequate vacuum devices and surgical masks, and observe fire precautions.

106. With all patients who are being seen for cosmetic treatments, make certain you spend time talking about the outcome and any limitations of the results.

107. For removing seborrheic keratoses, consider using cryotherapy followed by curetting.

108. Do not prescribe oral retinoid agents unless you are knowledgeable about proper administration and monitoring techniques.

109. Think of cryosurgery as controlled frostbite, not uncontrolled necrosis.

110. Make certain your elderly patients sit up slowly after undergoing a procedure.

111. For patients with tinea capitis, consider adding twice-weekly shampooing with 2% selenium sulfide for its sporicidal activity, which may prevent its spread to other children and family members.

112. Make certain you pull back on the syringe before you inject.

113. Ensure that all patients wear pressure bandages after leg vein injections.

114. Before you pick up a surgical tool, confirm that the operative consent form has been signed.

115. Patients should stop taking vitamin E before undergoing surgery.

Surgeons must be very careful—
When they take up the knife!
Underneath their fine incisions—
Stirs the Culprit—LIFE!

Emily Dickinson

116. Always repair a defect with the simplest closure possible.

117. Systemic infections, all kinds of stress, and the use of beta-blocking medications, antimalarial agents, and lithium can precipitate or exacerbate psoriasis.

118. Be careful to avoid the use of topical steroid medications on patients with perioral dermatitis.

119. *Trichophyton rubrum* causes more fungal diseases of the skin than any other fungal species.

120. In any patient who has a kerion, check for posterior cervical lymphadenopathy.

121. It is common to see improvement of hidradenitis suppurativa, rheumatoid arthritis, psoriasis, sarcoidosis, and atopic dermatitis during pregnancy.

122. Keep in mind the dermatologic emergencies, including pyoderma gangrenosum, dermatomyositis, bullous systemic lupus erythematosus (SLE), toxic epidermal necrolysis (TEN), and septicemia.

123. Most patients will have a pigmentation disorder during their lifetime.

124. Tell patients who have experienced pigment changes following an inflammatory episode that resolution to normal may take several months.

125. Consider giving topical steroid agents concurrently with patients undergoing treatment with 5-fluorouracil to reduce the severity of the irritation.

Tom Sawyer on curing warts:

You got to go all by yourself, to the middle of the woods, where you know there's a spunk-water stump, and just as it's midnight you back up against the stump and jam your hand in and say:

> *Barley-corn, barley-corn, injun-meal shorts,*
> *Spunk-water, spunk-water, swaller these warts,*

and then walk away quick, eleven steps, with your eyes shut, and then turn around three times and walk home without speaking to anybody. Because if you speak the charm's busted.

The Adventures of Tom Sawyer by Mark Twain

126. Don't forget sunlight in the treatment of psoriasis—and recommend using sun block on the appropriate places.

127. Biopsy all subungual warts in HIV-positive patients to rule out squamous cell carcinoma.

128. At times it is better to limit damage rather than cure.

Don't defy the diagnosis,
try to defy the verdict.

Norman Cousins

129. Most of medicine is a humbling business.

130. Above all else, do no harm!

131. If you worry about things that *might* happen, a lot of the things you worry about *won't* happen.

132. With a subungual hematoma, the pigment is confined to the nailbed and gradually grows out with the nail.

133. *Pseudomonas aeruginosa* is the most common cause of green nails (the bacterium produces a pycyanin pigment to the nail plate) and can be treated by cutting the nail away and applying antibiotic.

134. Arthropods (invertebrates that arise from eggs) such as scabies, lice, ants, and spiders are the most successful of all living animals (1 million named species), and they aren't going away soon!

135. Do not enter lightly into the world of retinoids, methotrexate, and cyclosporine when treating psoriasis.

136. Talk to associates who specialize in the treatment of arthritis when you are treating psoriasis patients who complain of aches, pains, and swelling of joints.

137. Elderly patients with poor ejection fractions do not tolerate long procedures well.

138. Good procedures and visits deserve good notes on the chart.

139. Check for allergies, antibiotic prophylaxis, and anticoagulants in all surgical patients.

140. Getting well means more to a patient than getting the diagnosis.

141. The goal of science is to build better mouse-traps; the goal of nature is to build better mice.

Medicine, the only profession that labours incessantly to destroy the reason for its existence.

James Bryce

142. Consider the use of itraconazole, topical steroid medications, antihistamines, and ultraviolet B phototherapy in treating patients with HIV-associated eosinophilic folliculitis.

143. Up to 5% of actinic keratoses will develop into squamous cell carcinomas, and a variety of treatments are available.

144. The guidelines for melanoma-prone families include frequent examinations, sun protection, and precautions regarding hormone therapy.

145. More than 90 topical steroid preparations are available in the United States—plan carefully and choose which vehicle and potency would work best.

146. Whenever possible, do not treat patients over the telephone.

147. Don't be overly optimistic concerning treatment or prognosis.

Nature, time, and patience are the three great physicians.

Proverb

148. In a patient who is doing well, don't just do something—stand there!

149. Keep Monsel's solution off the face to avoid staining.

150. Use oral antibiotic medications for patients with seborrheic dermatitis who have developed a secondary infection.

151. Look for necrotizing ear infections brought on by *Pseudomonas aeruginosa* in patients with diabetes.

Science without religion is lame;
religion without science is blind.

Albert Einstein

152. It is better to leave a little epidermis than to take too much of the dermis.

153. Never hesitate to redo a repair if you are not happy with it.

154. Just because you are a skin specialist doesn't mean you can't recommend weight loss for patients with acanthosis nigricans and exogenous obesity.

155. The young dermatologist knows of a dozen ways to treat a single disease; the old dermatologist knows a single way to treat a dozen diseases.

PATIENTS AND THEIR FAMILIES

Let the surgeon take care to regulate the whole regimen of the patient's life for joy and happiness. . . . Allow his relatives and special friends to cheer him up, and by having someone tell him jokes . . . keep up your patient's spirit by music and viols and ten-stringed psaltery. The surgeon must forbid anger, hatred and sadness in the patient, and remind him that the body grows fat from joy, and thin from sadness.

Henry de Mondeville, professor of surgery (1260-1320)

156. All patient care is less stressful if you are good at it.

157. The patient who badmouths his previous dermatologist and sings your praises will also turn on you in a split second.

158. Beware of patients with a list of ten problems at the initial consultation.

159. Someone who is rude to your receptionist and gives your nurse a hard time may not be the kind of patient you wish to get involved with.

160. Beware of the patient who has money for a skin care product but not his insurance co-payment.

161. Elderly patients are like potato chips: if handled roughly, they will crumble.

162. Talk to all your patients who smoke about quitting.

163. Verticality nourishes brevity, but sometimes it's good to just sit and talk with your patients.

164. Always knock before you enter an examination room and say goodbye when you leave.

165. Never blame a patient for his or her disease.

166. Be honest with patients about whether a procedure is curative or merely palliative.

To cure sometimes,
to relieve often,
to comfort always.

Anonymous

167. A minor procedure for you is still a major procedure for your patient.

168. Never make promises about results or outcomes.

169. When visiting with patients or families, sit down as if you had all day, even when you don't.

170. Conduct yourself in a dignified, professional manner.

171. The key to the care of patients is caring about your patients.

Treat people as if they were what they ought to be and you help them to become what they are capable of being.

Johann von Goethe

Looks are so deceptive that people should be done up like packages with the ingredients clearly labeled.

Helen Hudson

172. Be aware of an inadequate oral history and document.

173. Physicians lose their patients when they lose their patience.

174. It's nice to be important, but it's more important to be nice.

175. The number of side effects of a drug is directly proportional to the number known by the patient.

176. Be aware of patient personality types and treat each patient accordingly.

177. The three most important skills in medicine: listening, listening, and listening.

The reason we have two ears
and only one mouth
is that we may listen the more
and talk the less.

Zeno of Eleas, fifth-century bc Greek philosopher

178. When having a bad managed-care day, remember that managed care is not your patient's fault.

179. Be aware that your words can have a powerful emotional impact and influence.

180. Never, never make statements such as this: "Well, at least you don't have AIDS."

181. Don't think out loud or be self-critical in front of your patient.

182. Do not avoid the family of a patient who isn't doing well.

183. When you greet patients, look them in the eye.

184. Always have a hand mirror in each examination room for the patient to use when pointing out his or her problems to you.

185. Explain what you are doing, and the treatment's risks and benefits.

186. Discuss alternative treatments with your patient.

*Care more for
the individual patient than
for the special features
of the disease.*

Sir William Osler

187. Kill a nasty patient with kindness.

188. Never let a patient encounter pass without some physical contact.

The Human Touch

Tis the human touch in this world that counts,
The touch of your hand and mine
That means far more to the fainting heart
Than shelter, bread, or wine.
For the shelter is gone when the night is over
And bread only lasts for the day.
But the touch of a hand and the sound of a voice
Sing on in the soul always.

Spencer Michael Free

189. When dealing with a patient in the postoperative period, do the least in the greatest amount of time possible.

190. Always give the postoperative patient your home phone number. They'll think you're so nice, they would never dream of calling and disturbing you.

191. Maintain good communications with your patients.

192. Most malpractice suits are the result of poor communication between physicians and patients or families.

193. Be prompt and respectful of your patients.

194. Maintain patient confidences.

195. Document telephone complaints.

196. When a patient is not making progress, don't hesitate to seek another opinion; it may save you the embarrassment of having the patient request one first.

197. Realize that every patient has something to teach you.

It is much more important to know what sort of a patient has a disease than what sort of a disease a patient has.

Sir William Osler

198. Remember that all the points on a "learning curve" are real people with real lives.

199. Understand clearly the difference between what the patient needs and what the patient will tolerate.

200. Make a housecall on occasion—it's good to see the patient in his or her own milieu.

201. Your bedside manner is still your most valuable clinical skill.

202. Pay attention to medical articles in the popular press. These are what the patients and their families read.

203. Advise patients of test results and the need for follow-up appointments.

204. Don't refill prescriptions for topical medications if you want to see the patient again.

205. Your biggest responsibility at consultation is to explain things to the patient and family members in terms they can understand.

*Nothing in life is to be feared.
It is to only be understood.*

Marie Curie

*Only in the darkness of
self-deception can fear thrive;
fear cannot grow in the light of
questioning and understanding.*

Robert A. Norman

STAFF AND COLLEAGUES

It is beneficial to remember that the entire population of the universe, with one trifling exception, is composed of others.

John Andrew Holmes

206. Be as friendly as possible to everyone you meet—they could be the good source of referrals, or future patients.

207. Treat your technical sales representatives cordially; their jobs are important to them too.

208. If your office staff is not friendly and empathetic, you won't be successful.

209. Never let suntanned women work in your office.

210. Never badmouth a colleague in front of a patient or a patient's family—it makes you both look bad.

211. Consider it a great compliment when asked to care for a colleague or a colleague's family.

212. Remember that other people think their jobs are tough, too.

213. Understand the following translations:
"In my experience"—one case
"In case after case"—two cases
"In my series"—three or four cases

214. The New England Journal of Medicine reports that nine of ten doctors agree that one of ten doctors is an idiot.

The best index to a person's character is
(1) how he treats people who can't do him any good, and
(2) how he treats people who can't fight back.

Abigail Van Buren (Dear Abby)

215. Treat your colleagues as partners and your partners as colleagues.

216. Don't be harder on your team than you are on yourself.

I don't believe in just ordering people to do things. You have to sort of grab an oar and row them in.

Harold Geneen

217. Realize that your team watches *everything* you do.

218. No good deed goes unpunished.

219. Try to remember that the members of your team have lives, too.

220. Don't overlook the contribution that your secretary makes to the success of your practice.

221. Never assume an administrator knows more about your practice than you do.

222. Don't be critical of others until you have done a complete investigation of all relevant facts.

223. Be skeptical of the claims of colleagues who insist they *never* see a particular complication.

224. Learn to recognize the difference between colleagues who are physicians and those who are entrepreneurs with medical degrees.

225. Don't depend on anyone else to assign diagnostic codes to each case for you.

226. Disagree with your partners privately—support them publicly.

227. Referrals should not be looked on as gifts or favors, but rather as decisions that have been entrusted to you about the welfare of fellow human beings.

228. If a patient is referred to you, never belittle the care provided by the referring person.

229. Learn to quickly recognize when a referral really reflects someone's wanting his or her problem to become your problem.

230. If you find two colleagues you can really trust, you're twice as lucky as most.

231. Be wary of colleagues who are more familiar with their billings than they are with their results.

232. Never send your secretary to do your birthday or Christmas shopping.

233. Protect your assistants and surgical team members from blood exposure just as you would yourself.

234. Don't be overly influenced by those not as motivated and ambitious as you.

235. The difference between dermatologists and other physicians is that dermatologists wash their hands *before* going to the bathroom.

236. Calling the primary care physician of a patient with a serious problem shows good judgment, not weakness.

237. Do not flirt with your nurses or support staff.

238. Your younger partners should be able to teach you as well as learn from you.

239. How physicians at different levels read a scientific article:

• First-year resident	Reads entire article
• Senior resident	Reads abstract
• Chief resident	Reads author location and affiliation for job possibility
• Junior staff	Checks authors' names to see what peers are doing
• Senior staff	Checks references to see if quoted
• Emeritus staff	Doesn't read—published same findings years ago

240. Care for your partners' patients as enthusiastically as you do your own.

All things by immortal power,
Near or far
Hiddenly
To each other linked are,
That thou canst not stir a flower,
Without troubling a star.

Francis Thompson, 1897

PROFESSIONAL DEVELOPMENT

If you want to give God a good laugh, tell him your plans.

Yiddish folk saying

The basic difference between an ordinary man and a warrior is that a warrior takes everything as a challenge, while an ordinary man takes everything either as a blessing or a curse.

Don Juan

241. The advantage of dermatology as a career choice is that no one ever dies and no one ever gets better.

242. Remember that it's not only how you are with patients, but what you do when you're not in the office that makes you the kind of physician you are.

243. Know your limitations, preferably ahead of time.

244. If you act like one of the clowns, you will never run the circus.

245. Don't underestimate the power of media influence on the "science" of clinical practice.

246. You should know two ways to do just about everything.

Do what you can,
with what you have,
where you are.

Theodore Roosevelt

247. When faced with the choice between brilliance and common sense, choose common sense every time.

248. Beware of statistical data. They are like swimsuits—encouraging in their revelation, vital in their concealment.

249. The hardest part of putting together a clinical trial is coming up with a catchy acronym for it.

250. As unappealing as it may seem, you have to become involved with the politics of health care.

251. Always be kind to the institution that trained you.

252. A good week is one in which you have more cases than meetings.

253. If you are on a hospital committee, skip half the meetings. You will get a reputation for being busy, and you won't miss anything.

254. In a very difficult situation, never underestimate the power of persistence.

255. Practice long enough and you will probably see everything.

256. Even on your last day of practice, there will be something new to learn.

257. Don't try to be all things to all people.

258. You cannot outrun statistics.

259. It is possible to be skeptical without being cynical.

Use soft words and hard arguments.

English proverb

260. Confidence is essential; arrogance is deadly.

261. Take your work seriously, yourself less so.

262. About the time you get it all figured out, it is time to retire.

263. The better you are, the luckier you get.

*One thing I know:
the only ones among you
who will be truly happy are those
who will have sought and found
how to serve.*

Albert Schweitzer, M.D.

264. Learn to trust your instincts.

265. There is no substitute for experience.

266. Physicians who don't examine their mistakes are destined to repeat them.

267. It is good to learn from your mistakes, but better to learn from someone else's.

If you want the present to be different from the past, study the past.

Baruch Spinoza

268. It's OK not to know something, as long as you know where to look it up or where to find someone who does know.

269. Never underestimate your competition.

270. In most parts of the country, there are enough dermatology cases to go around; don't be greedy.

271. If you love your work but hate your job, it might be time to look elsewhere.

No person who is enthusiastic about his work has anything to fear from life.

Samuel Goldwyn

272. Make cost containment an ongoing process in your program.

273. Participate in continuous quality-improvement programs.

274. Attend meetings that have presentations, not advertisements.

275. Don't confuse advertising copy with clinical information.

276. Don't say "paradigm shift" more than once a year.

277. Even if you're not a frequent contributor, on-line discussion forums can be of great value.

278. The seven deadly sins of medical practice are these: greed, arrogance, greed, arrogance, greed, arrogance, and greed.

279. Keep your paperwork pile short enough so that it's not mistaken for a rock-climbing wall.

280. Be more impressed by how much you have to learn than by how much you know.

281. It is easy to become cocky; it is hard to stay that way.

282. An arrogant attitude and a limited knowledge base form a dangerous combination.

283. Look critically at your results; everyone else will.

284. A certain amount of paranoia is healthy—whoever your "they" might be, they are out to get you.

285. Keep your mind and your desk as clean as possible.

286. Document your practice—appointments, medical records, prescriptions, correspondence, and communications.

287. Beware of managed-care overload—the skin needs experts who are not interested in how the fees are paid.

288. Don't ever alter a patient's records; your job is to doctor the patient, not doctor the records.

289. Completing your medical records in a timely manner is a responsibility, not a favor.

290. Beware of "entangling alliances" with pharmaceutical and equipment vendors.

291. To avoid a breach of contract, be careful about trying to maintain a specific result.

292. Remember that for medicolegal purposes, if it's not in the chart, it didn't occur.

293. Never forget—lawyers are sharks and you are dinner.

294. Forgive litigious attorneys, but write down their names.

295. It is impossible not to take a lawsuit personally.

296. Malpractice litigation is usually less about right and wrong than it is about moving money around.

297. Take time to read the nurse's notes; the lawyers certainly will.

298. Avoid even the appearance of professional conflict of interest.

299. Don't take on more work than you can effectively and efficiently cover.

For peace of mind, resign as general manager of the universe.

Larry Eisenberg

300. At some time in your career, review the world literature on *something.*

301. Join and actively support at least one medical organization.

302. Manage change graciously.

A sense of humor can help you
overlook the unattractive,
tolerate the unpleasant,
cope with the unexpected, and
smile through the unbearable.

Moshe Waldoks

303. Laugh at yourself.

A cheerful heart is a good medicine,
but a downcast spirit dries up the bones.

Proverbs 17:22

304. Embrace creativity—brainstorm constantly, experiment fearlessly, and adopt new ideas when they serve the interests of your practice.

305. Practice "right-jobbing"—make certain you and your staff members are each doing what you do best.

306. Maintain your *GASGMP*—*g*radually *a*ccepted *s*tandards of *g*ood *m*edical *p*ractice.

307. You're only as good as your last case.

308. Keep in mind the three *A*'s of a successful practice: be able, be affable, and be available.

309. Know how to use a personal computer for more than games and e-mail.

310. Life is short—buy a fast computer.

311. Never own a pager that is smarter than you are.

312. More important than having a great idea is recognizing a great idea.

313. There is no such thing as an uninteresting patient, only an uninterested physician.

314. Know yourself; schedule your toughest cases in the morning if that's when you have the most energy and attention.

315. Make certain you are comfortable before doing any procedure.

In the field of observations,
chance favors the prepared mind.

Louis Pasteur

316. Your medical records are a representation of the quality of care you provide.

317. Try to enjoy doing dermatology as much as you enjoy being a dermatologist

Each day we have a right
To the comfort of the early morning light,
The beacon on life's shore
Promising one more, one more.

Robert A. Norman

Experience is not
what happens to a man.
It is what a man does with
what happens to him.

Aldous Huxley

PERSONAL DEVELOPMENT

I have often found that my solitude is a thing to love, to cherish, not just because of the absence of distractions from other people, but from the inward travels that it allows, unhindered from the noise of the outside world.

Robert A. Norman

You grow up the day you have the first real laugh at yourself.

Ethel Barrymore

318. While seeing patients, doing paperwork, and running your practice, don't forget to live.

319. Retirement planning should begin the day you enter practice.

320. Start funding your children's education as soon as possible.

321. Don't take journals with you on vacations.

322. Surprise your children by picking them up at school once in a while.

323. Don't behave badly just because you can.

324. You can't possibly read enough.

325. Never write checks your curriculum vitae can't cash.

326. Have a will drawn up—you only *think* you're immortal.

327. Don't take life too seriously; you'll never get out of it alive

Strength is not the absence of weakness but how we wrestle with our weaknesses.

Noah Benshea

328. One hundred years from now, it won't matter what kind of house you lived in, or what kind of car your drove, but only if you made a difference in the lives of others.

329. Realize early on that you cannot make enough money to compensate for an unhappy home.

330. Cut your own lawn; it is very therapeutic.

331. Your attitude determines your altitude.

Life is an adventure in forgiveness.

Norman Cousins

Life is God's novel. Let him write it.

Isaac Bashevis Singer

332. Try not to measure your worth by your W-2.

333. Undertake community service.

If I am not in my own behalf,
who will be in my behalf?
And if I am not for myself only,
what am I?
And if not in the present,
when?

Hillel, Jewish sage, first century BC to AD

334. Anything pleasurable in life is either illegal, immoral, or fattening, and everything not fitting into these categories causes cancer in rats.

335. The three G's of a long, happy life—go, give, and goof off.

336. Avoid the pursuit of meaningless midlife trophies.

337. Time may be a great healer—but a bad beautician.

*I don't think of all the misery,
but of all the beauty that
still remains.*

Anne Frank

338. Temper is like a nuclear weapon; its potential use can be as effective as and less damaging than its actual display.

339. The only thing that doesn't slow down as you get older is the rate at which everything doesn't slow down.

340. If your number of ex-spouses exceeds your number of ex-partners, you have a serious problem.

341. Remember that no dermatologist on his or her deathbed ever wished that they'd worked a little more.

342. In the long run, your accomplishments as a parent or a spouse will far outweigh anything you do in your clinical practice.

343. Keep smiling! Unrelenting stress *will* ultimately kill you.

To laugh often and much,
to win the respect of intelligent people
and the affection of children . . .
to leave the world a little better . . .
to know even one life has
breathed easier because you have lived,
that is to have succeeded.

Ralph Waldo Emerson